ME

My name is_____.

I am_____years old. Today is_____.
(Date)

My birthday is_____.

My favorite TV show is_____.

My favorite day is_____.

My favorite animal is_____.

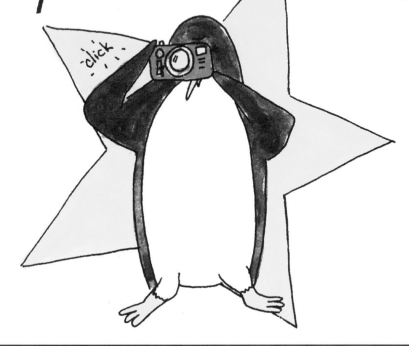

Place a photo
of yourself
here!

The person in my family who has cancer is_____.
(my brother, my mom, my aunt, me etc...)

When I found out it was cancer, I felt_____.

These are some things I know about cancer.

_____

_____

_____

_____

_____

_____

cancer?

These are some questions I would like to ask about cancer.

_____

_____

_____

_____

_____

_____

Life Isn't Always A Day At The Beach

A Book for *All* Children Whose Lives Are Affected By Cancer

Written by Pam Ganz
Illustrated by Tobi Scofield

If you are a school age child dealing with a diagnosis of cancer, this book is for you; maybe you or your sibling, parent or grandparent, relative or friend has been diagnosed with cancer. This diagnosis of cancer may cause many changes and adjustments in your life. It can be a difficult time for you as well as for family and friends. We hope that *Life Isn't Always A Day At The Beach* will help you cope with cancer by helping you express and share some of the many feelings and thoughts you may have. You may also understand your feelings better after writing, drawing or talking about them with a parent, family member, counselor, teacher or friend.

We chose a penguin for our book because children coping with cancer have a few things in common with penguins. Penguins are "different," they endure difficulties, and they need others for support. Now that cancer is a part of your life, you may feel different from others. Penguins, too, are different. Although penguins are birds, they are unlike other birds because they cannot fly in the air. However, penguins are Olympic swimmers and can "fly" in the water at speeds up to 30 mph using their wings as flippers.

When the female Emperor penguin lays her egg, the male will sit on it, keeping it warm for 65 days without eating, enduring the harsh weather of the Antarctic winter where the temperature may drop as low as -70°F. In addition, Chinstrap penguins often have to endure a long, difficult journey climbing over steep, rocky slopes to find food. Although these penguins encounter and endure such difficulties, they never give up. You, too, will face difficulties when dealing with cancer and we want to help you find your own special ways to endure.

Just as Emperor penguins rally together and huddle into a close group during a blizzard to stay warm, you can ask others to help you deal with cancer. Know that you are not alone. Others share your feelings and there are people willing to listen.

A Word to Adults . . .

- *Life Isn't Always A Day At The Beach* is intended to be used primarily with school age children ages 5–12, although older children have enjoyed using the book as well.

- The book was designed to be used with little or no adult guidance. However, younger children may need assistance with writing.

- All children can benefit from encouragement and support.

- Wait to offer help with brainstorming ideas until the child requests your help.

- Remember, this is the child's book. Let the child decide what to draw or write. Avoid making suggestions.

- Although the pages are numbered, there's no need to complete the pages in a particular order.

- The writings and drawings of the child will reflect their level of understanding about cancer and its treatment, their feelings, their hopes and concerns.

- It is our hope that *Life Isn't Always A Day At The Beach* will open avenues of communication between children and adults.

This is a drawing of my family before cancer.

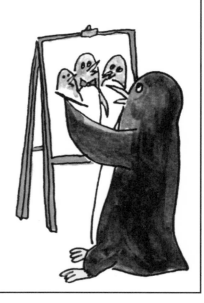

This is a drawing of my family now (after cancer).

Things I like to do with my family are
_____, _____ and _____.
This is my drawing of my favorite thing I like to do with my family:

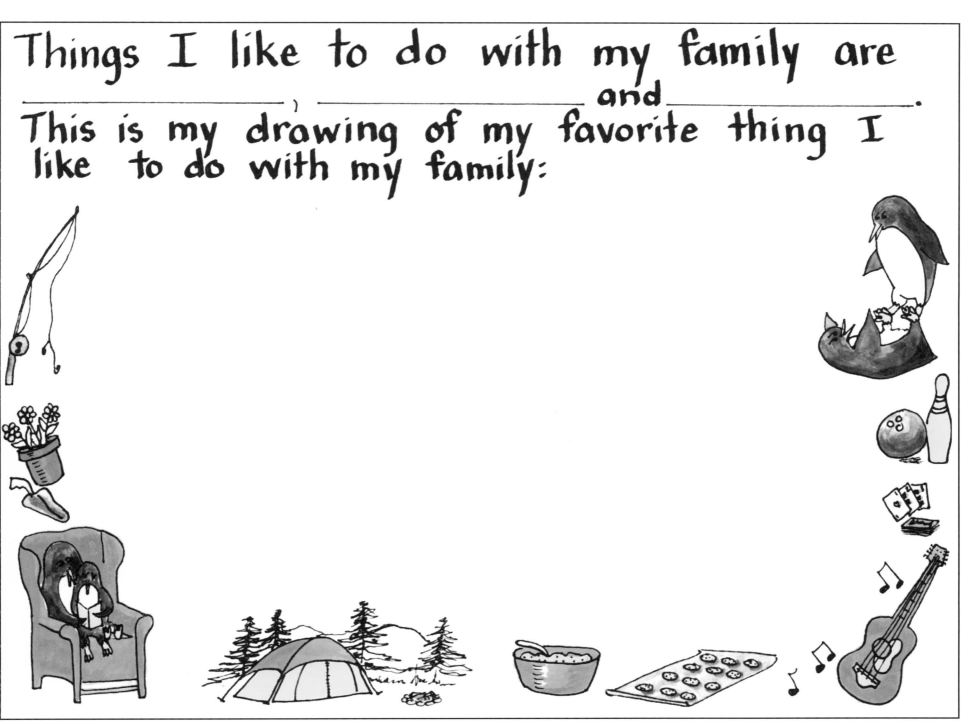

GOING TO THE HOSPITAL OR CLINIC

The best thing is_____
_____.

The worst thing is_____
_____.

This is a drawing of the hospital or clinic.

This is my drawing of the perfect hospital room.

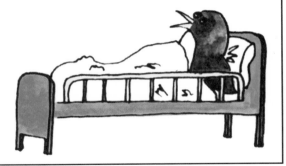

Treatment For Cancer

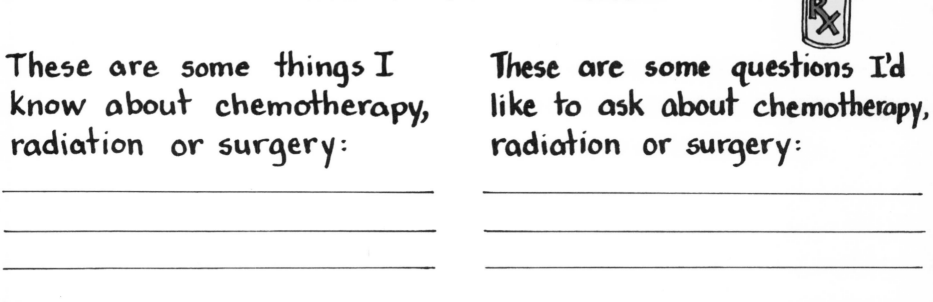

These are some things I know about chemotherapy, radiation or surgery:

_____
_____
_____
_____

These are some questions I'd like to ask about chemotherapy, radiation or surgery:

_____
_____
_____

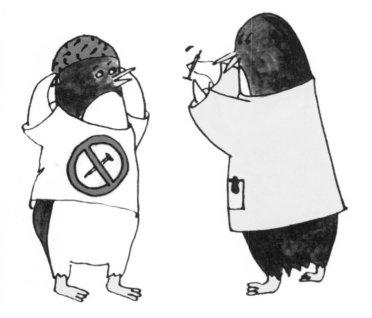

The hardest part of treatment is...

_____
_____
_____
_____
_____

I like it when the doctor(s)_____
_____,
I like it when the nurse(s)_____
_____,

If I could create the perfect medicine,
this is how it would work:

_____
_____
_____
_____
_____
_____
_____

If I could, I would put the cancer in a rocket and send it to_____.

This is my drawing of it going to_____.

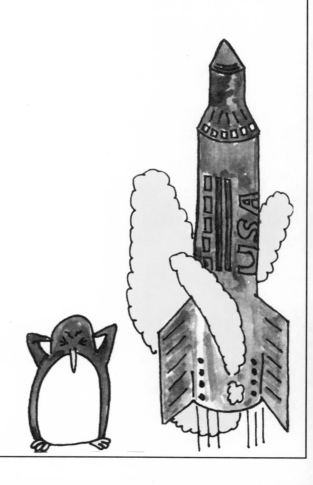

10

Cancer has changed some things in my life.

It seems unfair_____
_____.

I miss_____
_____.

I wish I could_____

Not all changes are bad.

Living with cancer has made me more_____
_____.

I appreciate_____more than I used to.

11

Sometimes I feel different because...

_____

_____

_____

These are some things I wish people understood about me:

_____   _____

_____   _____

_____   _____

_____   _____

Here are 5 great things about me.

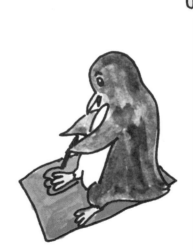

Trace around your hand and write something you like about yourself on each finger.

Living with cancer can feel like riding a roller coaster. There are <u>ups</u> and <u>downs</u>.

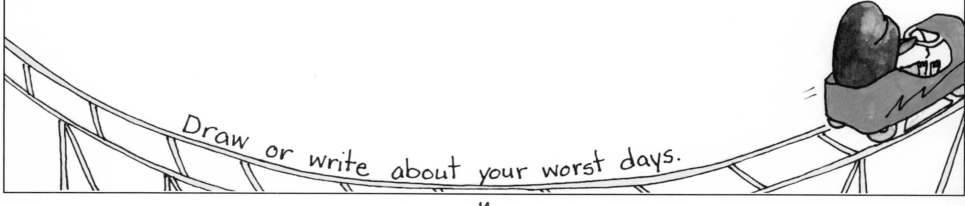

Draw or write about your worst days.

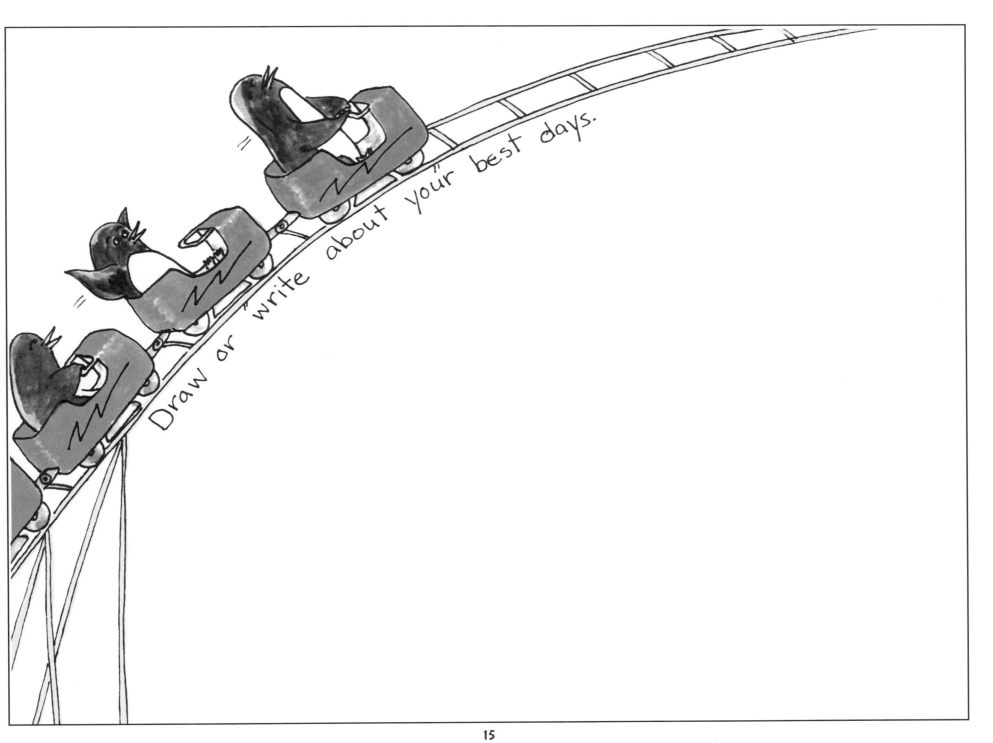

Draw or write about your best days.

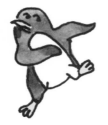 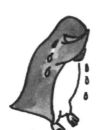 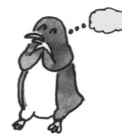 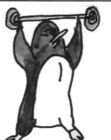 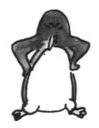 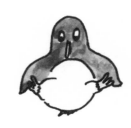

Sometimes I think my brother(s) or sister(s) feel_____because_____

_____

_____.

Sometimes I think my mom or dad feel_____because_____

_____

_____.

Sometimes I feel_____because_____

_____

_____.

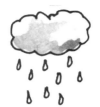

Feeling Sad

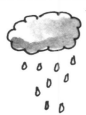

These are things that make me sad:

_____   _____

_____   _____

_____   _____

These are things I can do to help me when I'm sad. I can...

_____   _____

_____   _____

_____   _____

Feeling Angry

These are things that make me angry:

_____   _____

_____   _____

_____   _____

_____   _____

These are things I can do to help me
when I'm angry. I can...

_____   _____

_____   _____

_____   _____

_____   _____

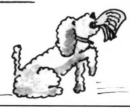

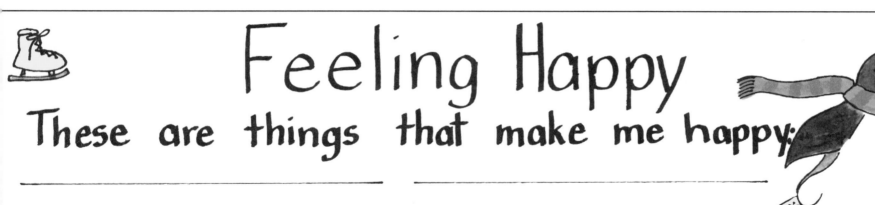

Feeling Happy

These are things that make me happy:

_____   _____

_____   _____

_____   _____

This is a drawing of me doing something
that makes me smile.

Feeling Scared

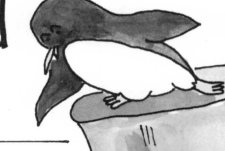

These are things I'm afraid of:

_____   _____

_____   _____

_____

> Drawing or talking about things you are afraid of can help take the fears away.

This is a drawing of something I'm afraid of.

Worries

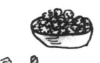

I worry about_____

_____

_____.

It helps to share worries with someone.

These are the people I can share my worries with:

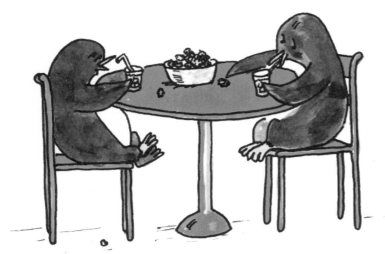

_____

_____

_____

_____

_____

School

The 3 best things about school are:

1._____
2._____
3._____

The 3 worst things about school are:

1._____
2._____
3._____

It helps me when my teachers_____

_____

_____.

It helps me when my classmates_____

_____

_____.

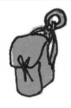

The hardest part about dealing with cancer and going to school is...

_____

_____

_____

_____

_____

Some questions my classmates have asked me about cancer are...

_____

_____

_____

_____

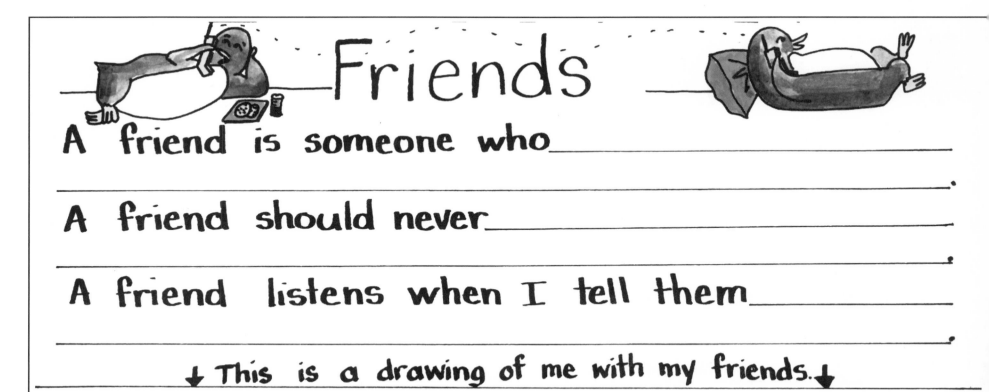

Friends

A friend is someone who_____
_____.

A friend should never_____
_____.

A friend listens when I tell them_____
_____.

↓ This is a drawing of me with my friends. ↓

Three Wishes

I wish my friends_____

_____

_____.

I wish my teachers_____

_____

_____.

I wish my parents_____

_____

_____.

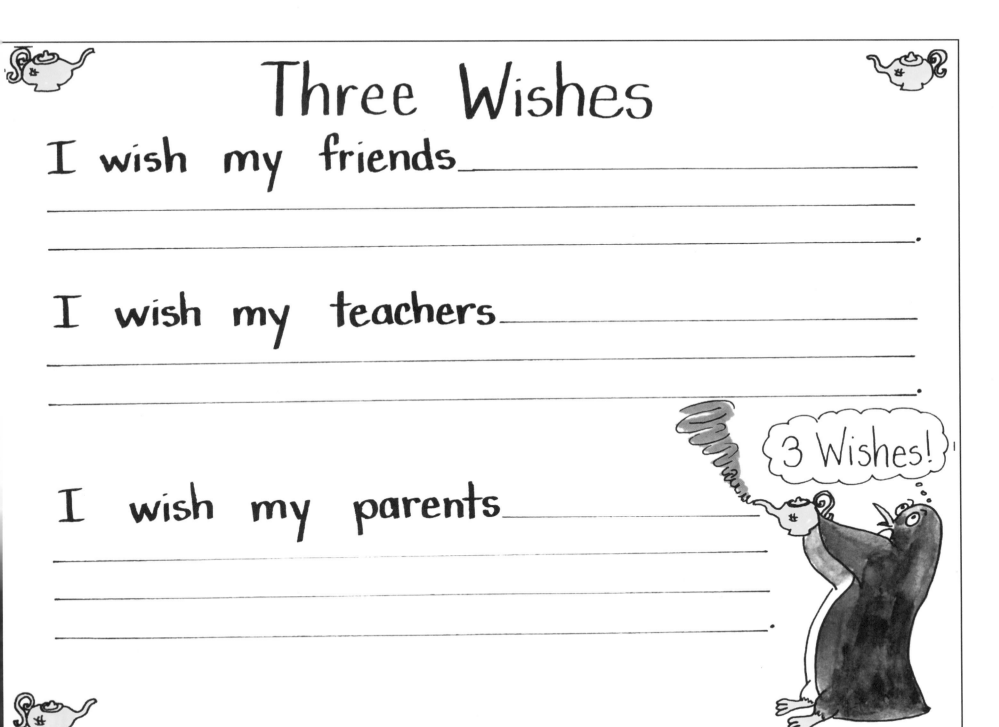

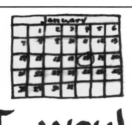

Future Plans

I would like to go_____

_____

_____

_____.

I would like to be_____

_____

_____.

I would like to see_____

_____

_____.

I would like to meet_____

_____.

_____.

Draw a picture of a rainbow and what you'd like to find at the end of your rainbow.

Create Your Own Page!

Use the following order form to receive more copies of *Life Isn't Always A Day At The Beach.*

High Five Publishing
Order Form

Quantity	Price Per Copy	Quantity Ordered	Subtotal *	Shipping and Handling	Total
1–11 copies	$9.95	×	=	+ $2.75	
12–24 copies	$8.95	×	=	+ $4.25	
25–79 copies	$7.95	×	=	+ $7.25	
80+ copies	$6.50	×	=	+ $10.50	
Nebraska residents add 6.5% sales tax to subtotal				**Total Enclosed**	

Shipping Address (Please Print)

Name_____

Organization _____

Street_____

City, State, Zip_____

Telephone _____

Foreign Country _____

For orders outside the U.S.A. shipping and handling charges
will be 10% of the subtotal, with a $2.75 minimum charge.

All orders must be prepaid in U.S. funds by check or money order. Make checks payable to High Five Publishing. For inquiries, our phone number is (402) 489-6060. Mail your order to:

High Five Publishing
4030 South 31st Street
Lincoln, Nebraska 68502

Allow 2–3 weeks for delivery. Orders outside the USA may take up to six weeks.
Thank you for your order.